FERNANDO L. PEROTTONI

BALDIES

A FIELD GUIDE TO THE NORTHERN HEMISPHERE

WORKMAN PUBLISHING, NEW YORK

Copyright © 2017 by Fernando L. Perottoni

All rights reserved. No portion of this book may be reproduced—mechanically, electronically, or by any other means, including photocopying—without written permission of the publisher. Published simultaneously in Canada by Thomas Allen & Son Limited.

Library of Congress Cataloging-in-Publication Data is available.

ISBN 978-0-7611-8915-2

Design by Ariana Abud

Workman books are available at special discounts when purchased in bulk for premiums and sales promotions as well as for fund-raising or educational use. Special editions or book excerpts also can be created to specification. For details, contact the Special Sales Director at the address below, or send an email to specialmarkets@workman.com.

Workman Publishing Co., Inc.
225 Varick Street
New York, NY 10014-4381
workman.com

WORKMAN is a registered trademark of Workman Publishing Co., Inc.

Printed in Hong Kong

First printing April 2017

10 9 8 7 6 5 4 3 2 1

> "There's many a man
> hath more hair than wit."
>
> *The Comedy of Errors* (act 2, scene 2)

———————————

Welcome to the Baldness Hall of Fame and Infamy—
an illustrated collection featuring some of the world's
most distinguished and distinguishable heads.

If you, reader, are part of this respected
and powerful group, count yourself lucky.

And if not, you are nonetheless invited to enjoy this
visual celebration of recognizably receding hairlines,
curious chrome domes, and peculiar pates.

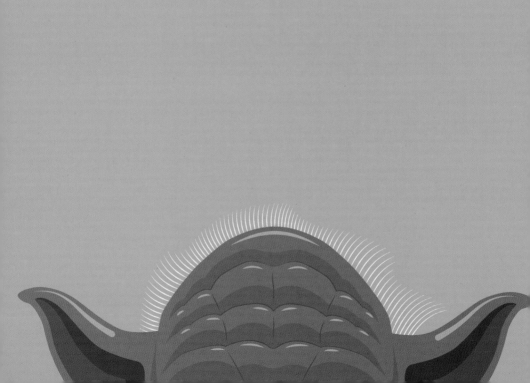

"When nine hundred years old you reach, look as good you will not."

"Guys are always patting my bald head for luck."

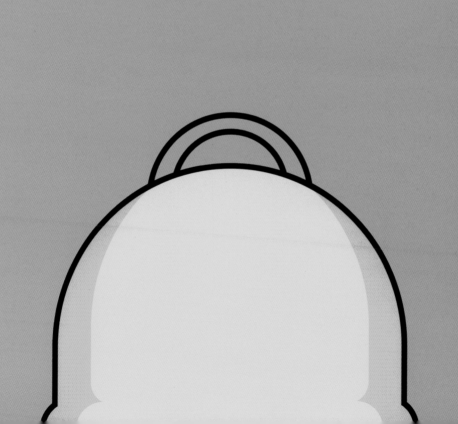

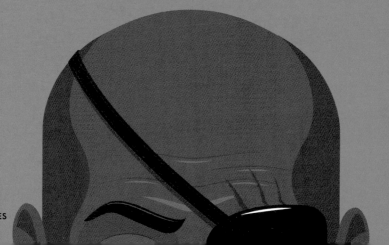

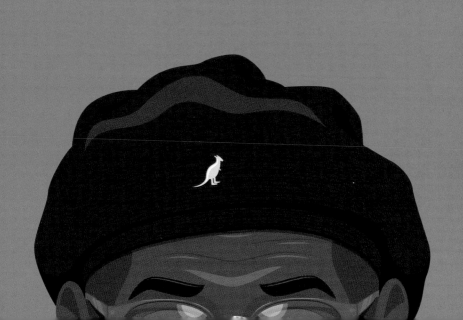

"Here's some simple advice:
Always be yourself.
Never take yourself too seriously.
And beware of advice from
experts, pigs, and members
of Parliament."

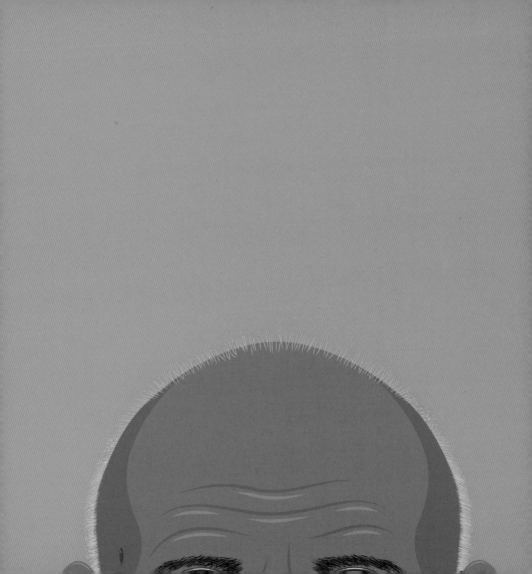

"Happiness is when what
you think, what you say, and what
you do are in harmony."

"I suppose I am a real professor, aren't I? Next thing you know, I'll be going bald."

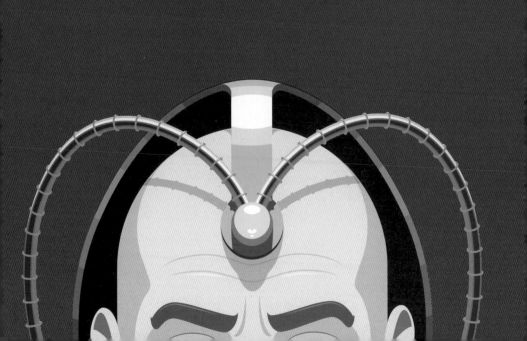

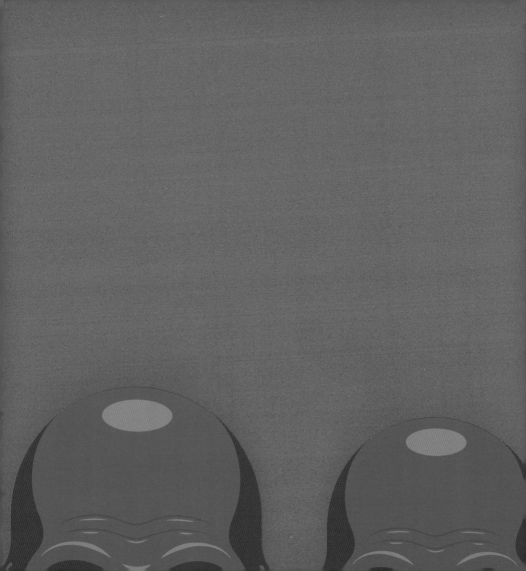

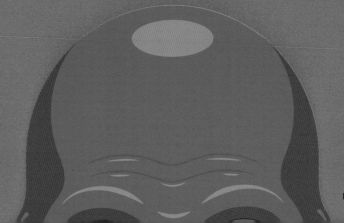

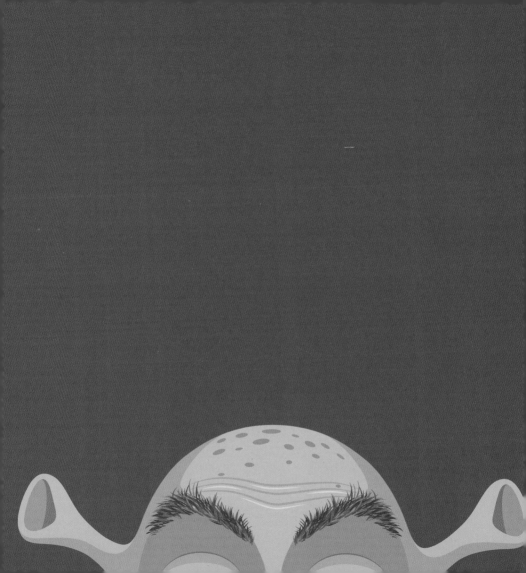

"Oh, you were expecting
Prince Charming?"

"There is much to be learned from beasts."

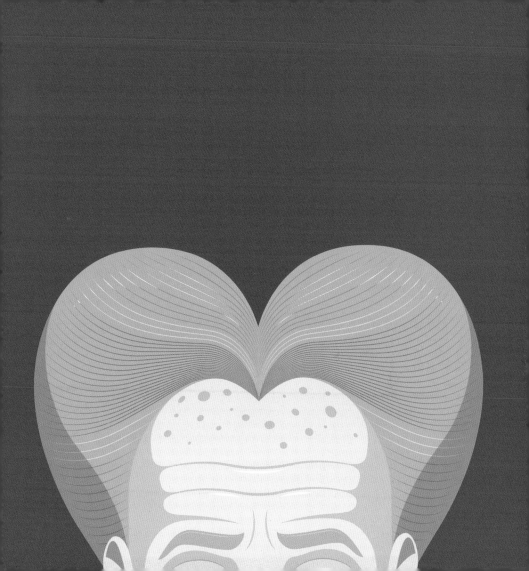

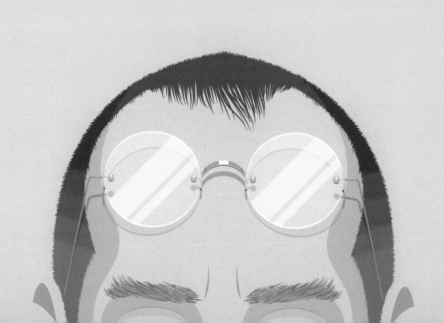

"Stay hungry.
Stay foolish."

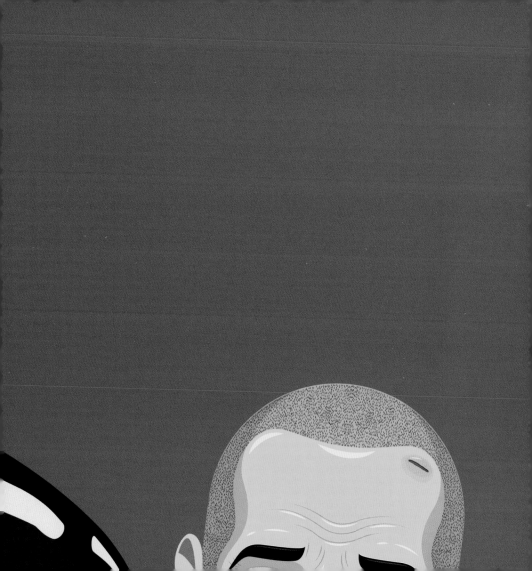

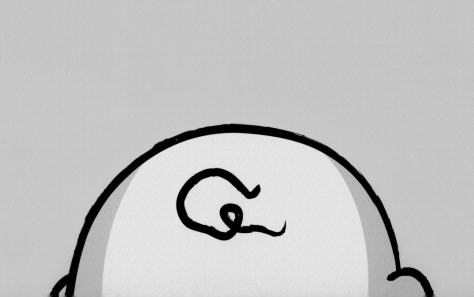

"I've developed a new philosophy . . .
I only dread one day at a time."

"Well, I wasn't a model student, but imagine being a bald fourteen-year-old in an elite prep school."

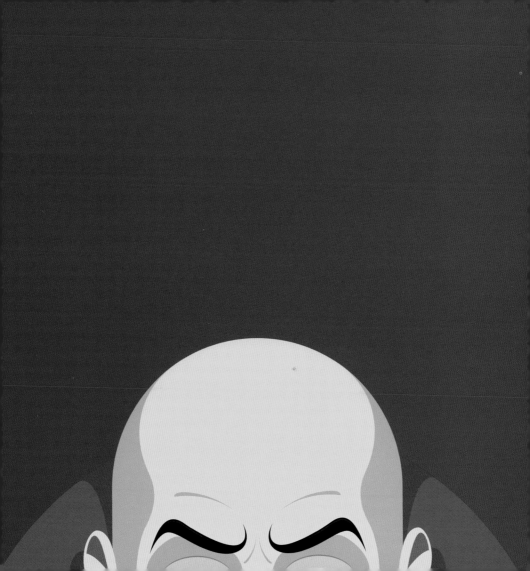

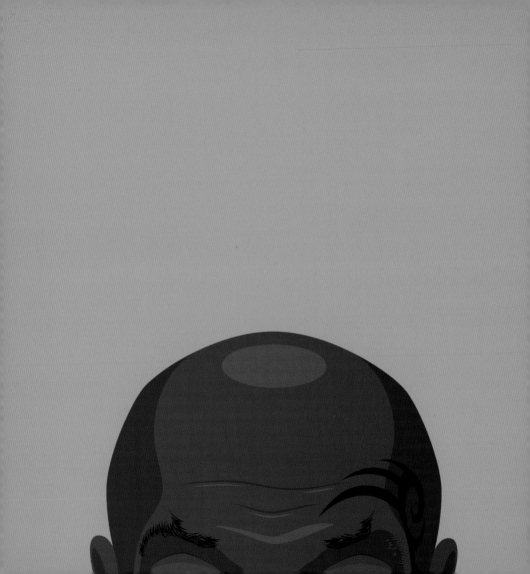

"Everybody has a plan until they get punched in the mouth."

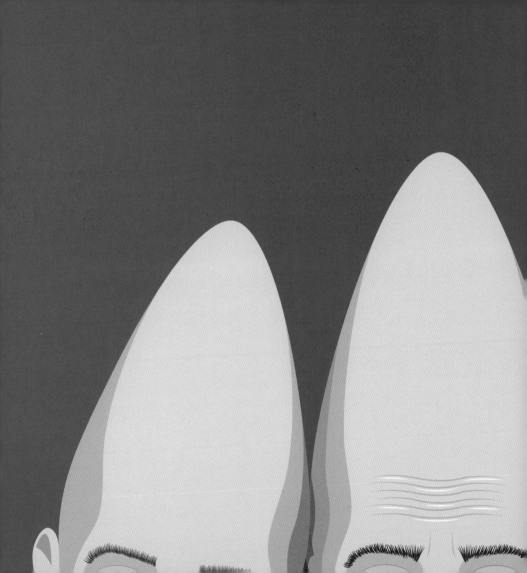

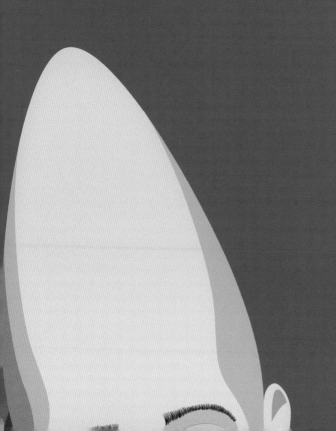

"Say my name."

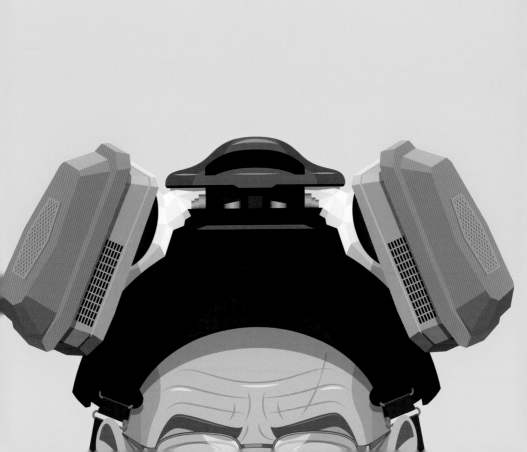

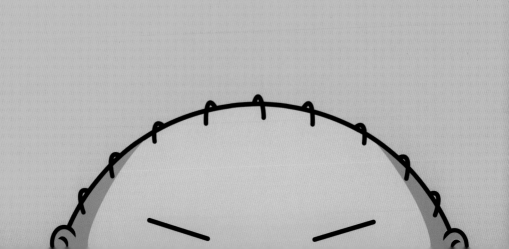

"What the deuce?"

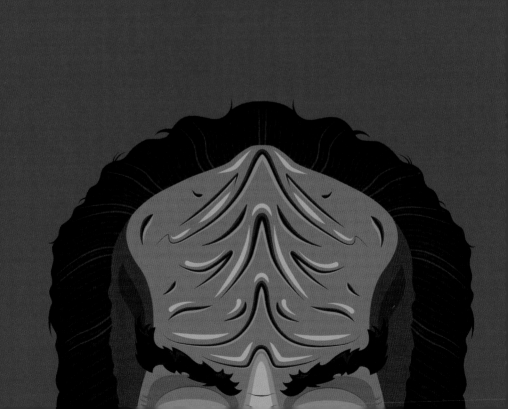

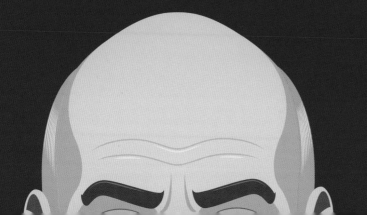

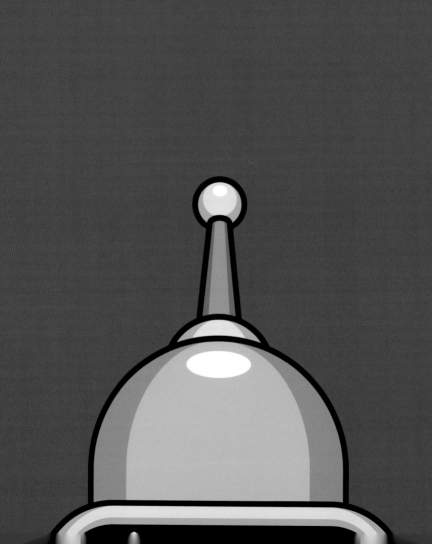

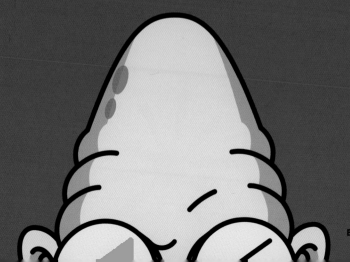

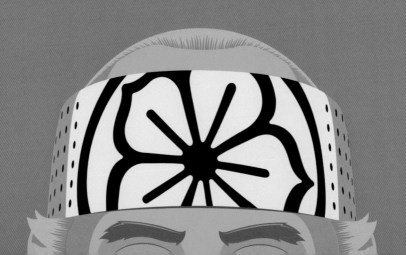

"Wax on, wax off."

"Painting is self-discovery.
Every good artist paints what he is."

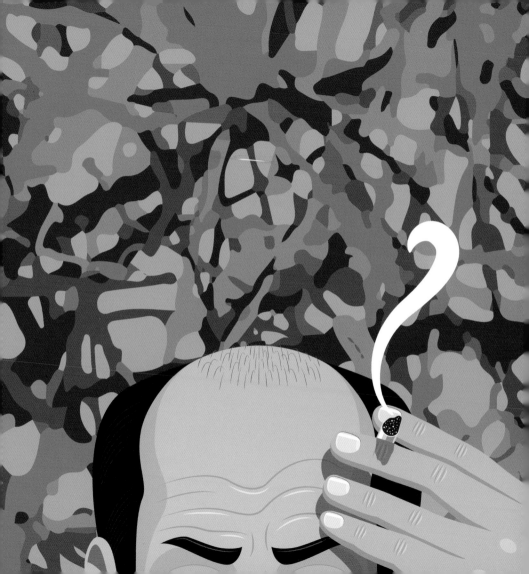

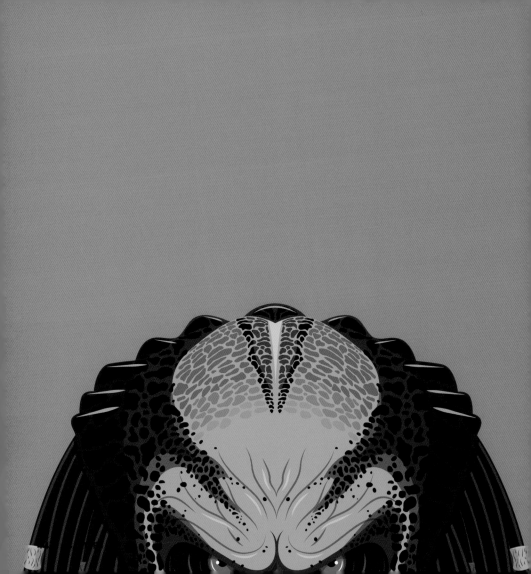

"What the hell are *you?*"

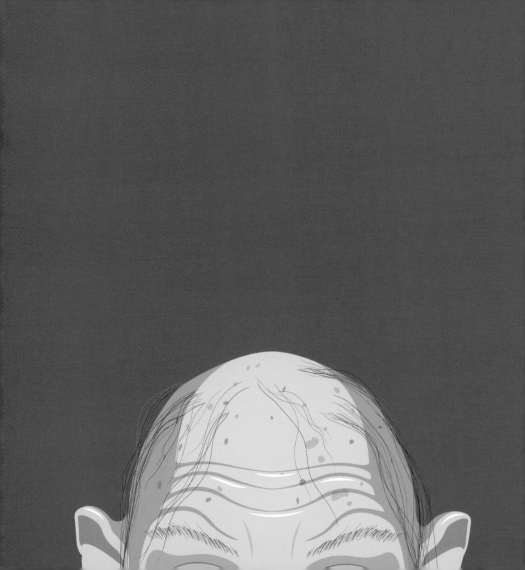

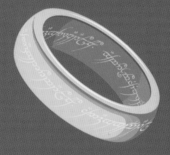

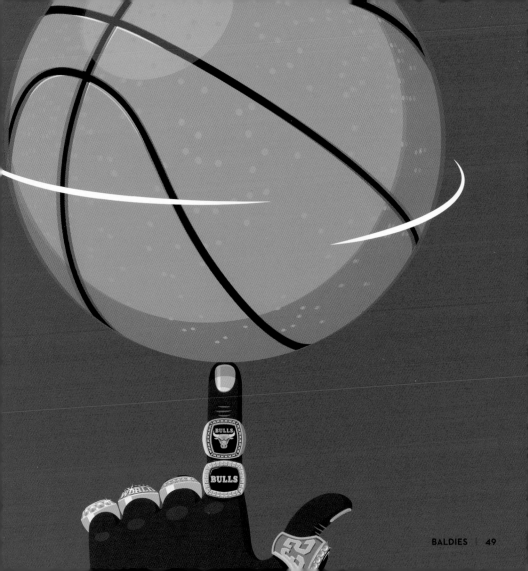

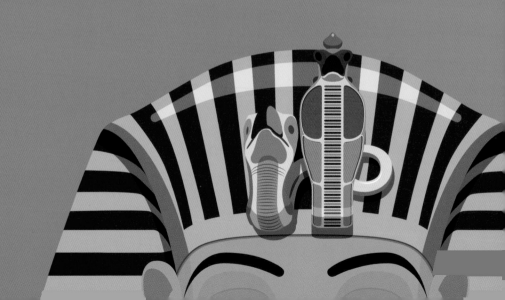

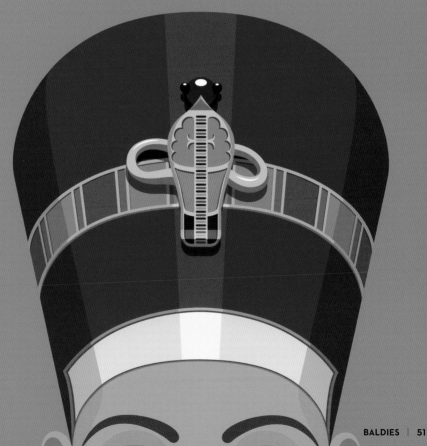

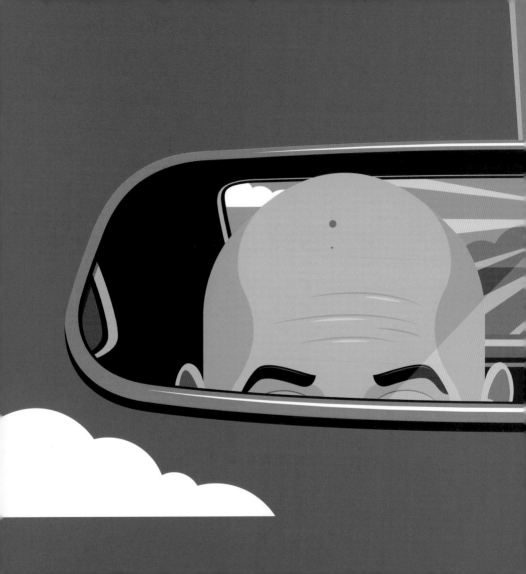

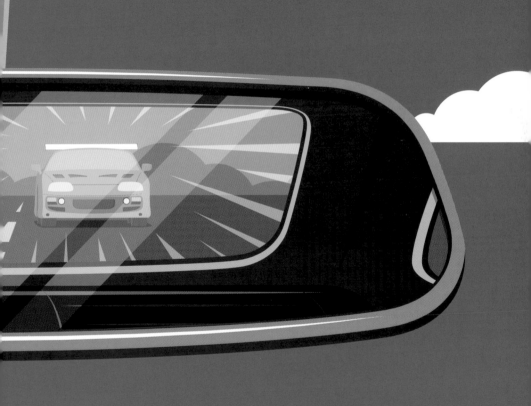

"You were good, kid, real good. But as long as I'm around, you'll always be second best, see?"

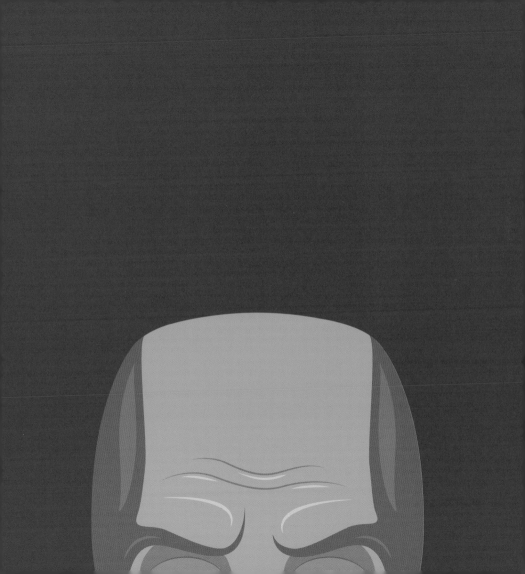

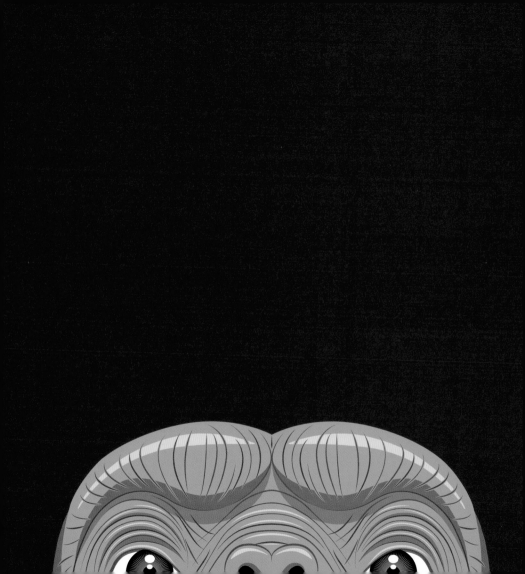

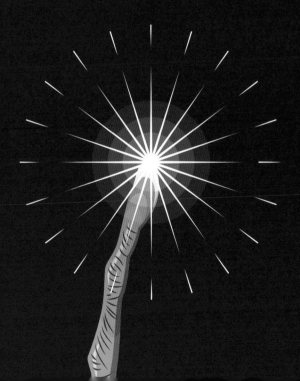

"Hey, believe me, baldness
will catch on. When the aliens come,
who do you think they're gonna relate to?
Who do you think is going to be the first
ones getting a tour of the ship?"

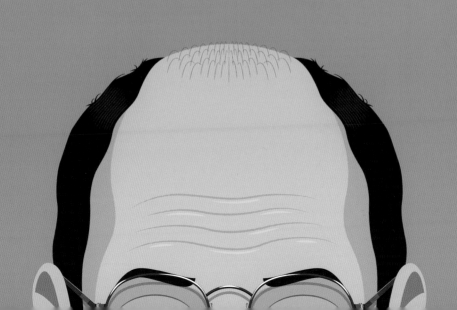

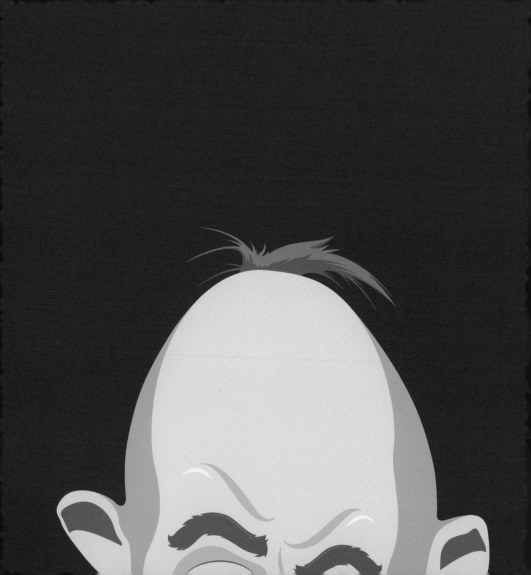

"Hey, you guys!"

"No. *I* am your father."

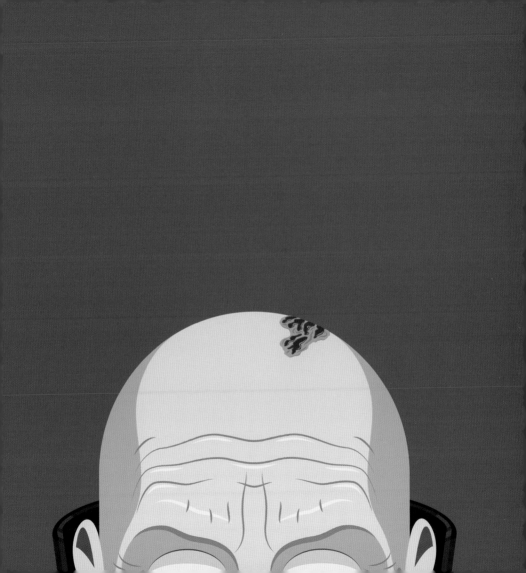

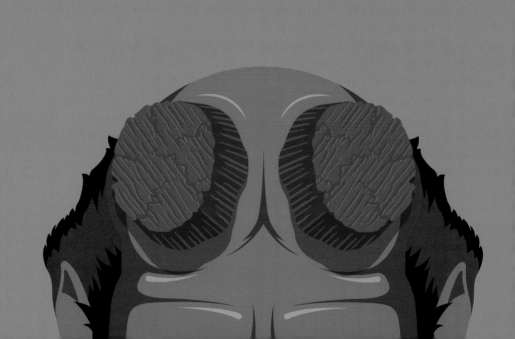

"I can promise you two things. One: I'll always look this good. Two: I'll never give up on you . . . ever."

"... We shall let the reader answer this question for himself: Who is the happier man, he who has braved the storm of life and lived or he who has stayed securely on shore and merely existed?"

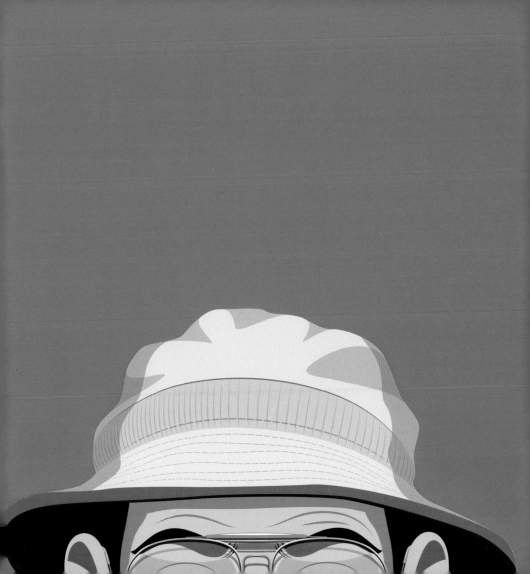

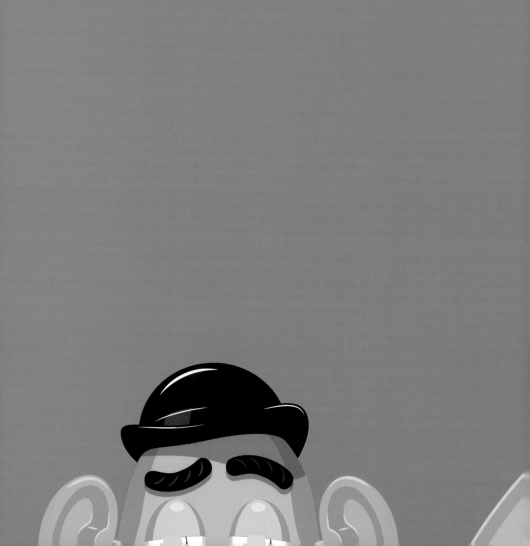

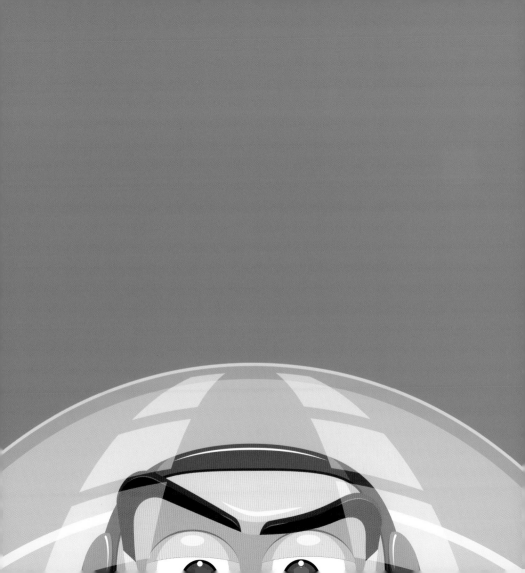

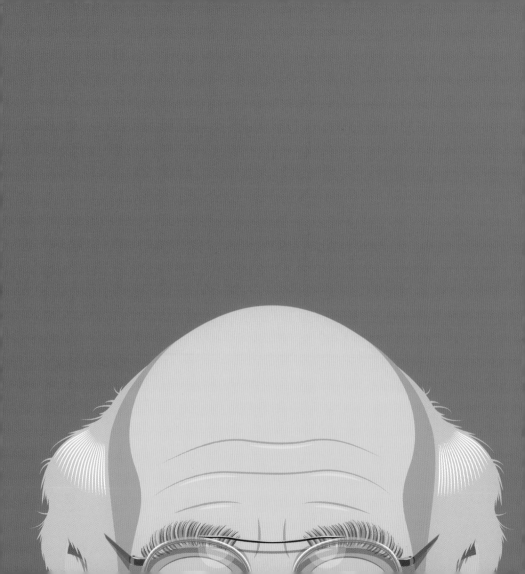

"Women love a self-confident bald man."

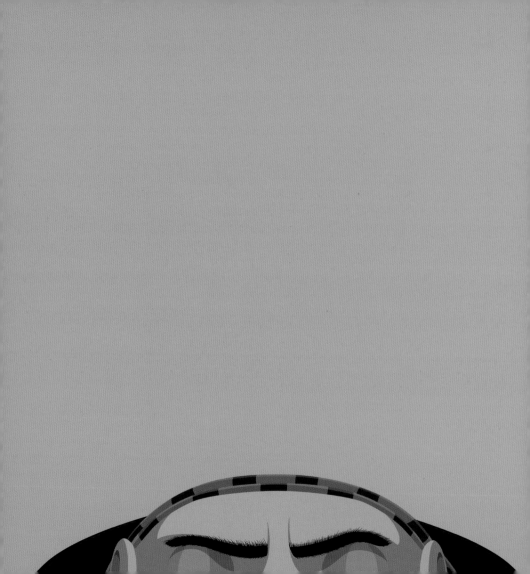

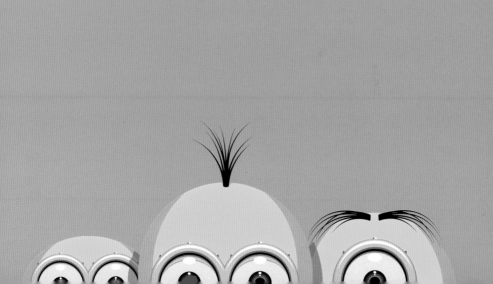

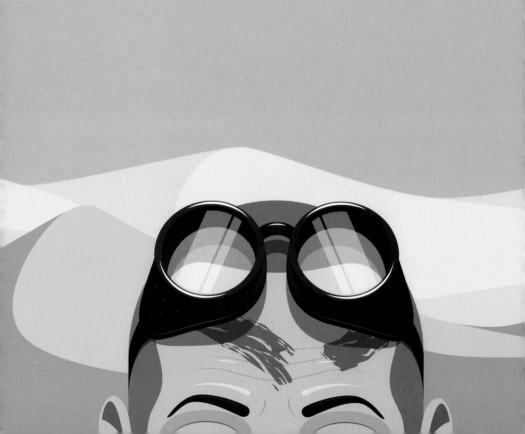

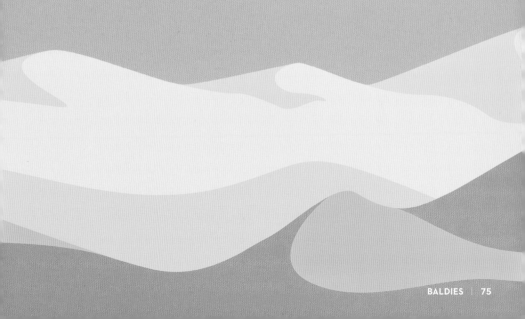

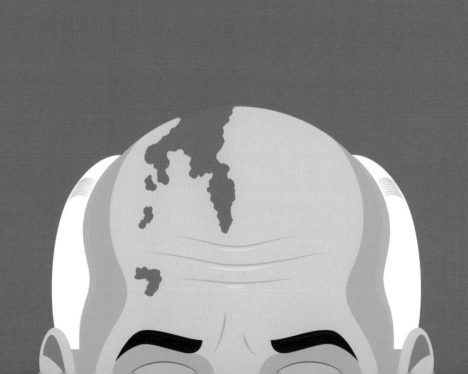

"If what you have done yesterday still looks big to you, you haven't done much today."

"This is your last chance.
After this, there is no turning back."

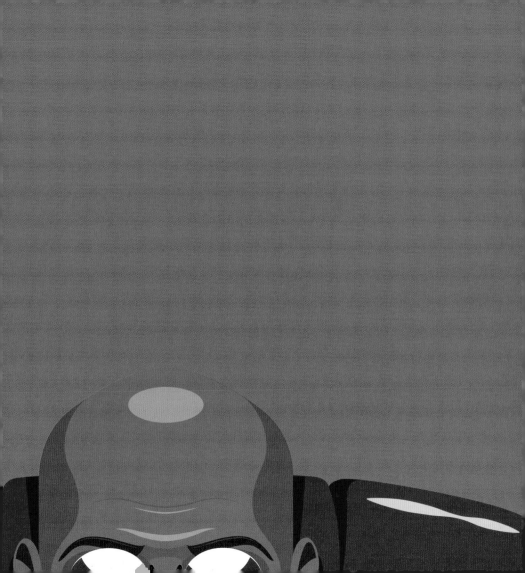

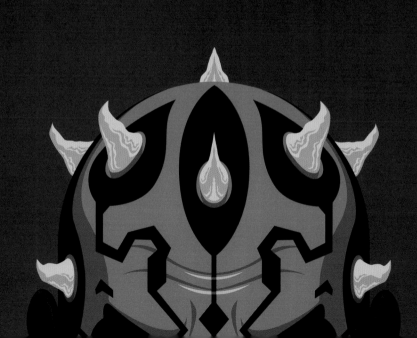

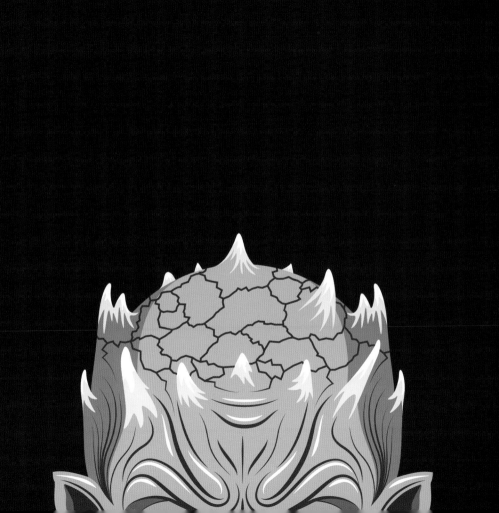

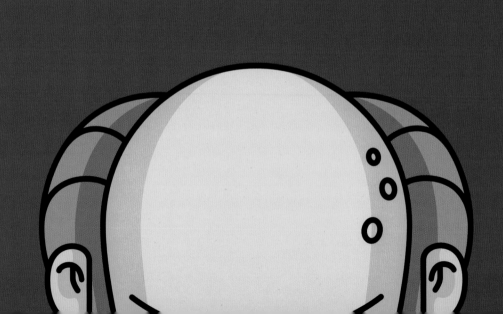

"Well, for once, the rich white man is in control."

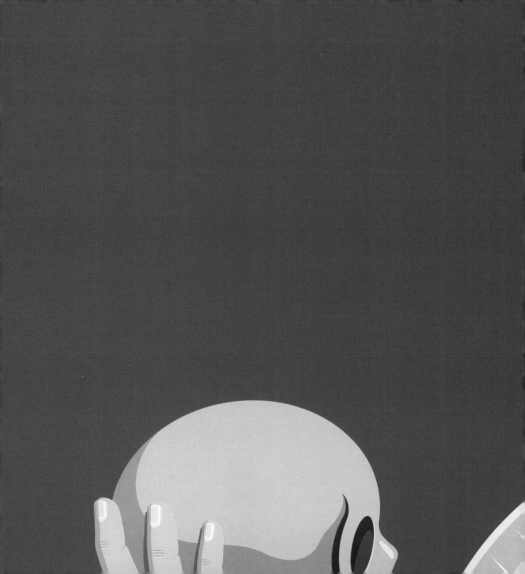

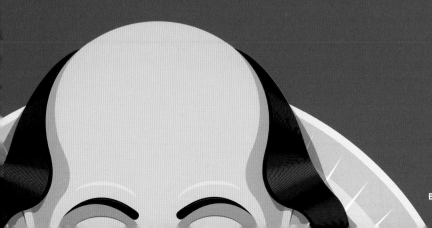

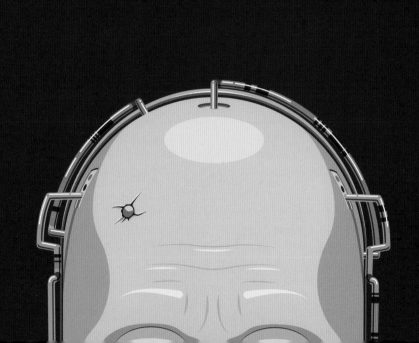

"Serve the public trust,
protect the innocent,
uphold the law."

"Yeah. That is a gun in my pants. But that doesn't mean I'm not happy to see you . . ."

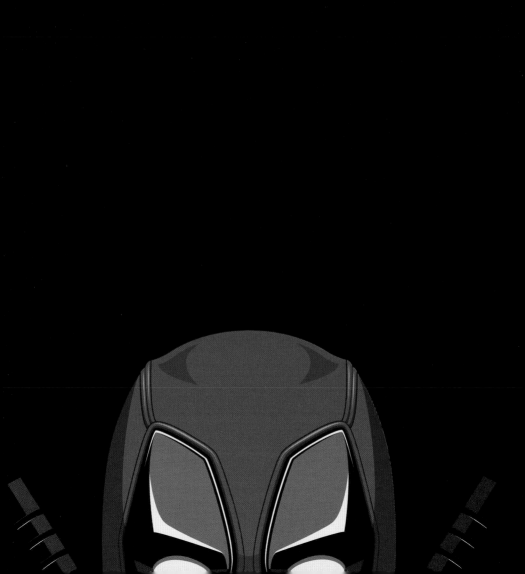

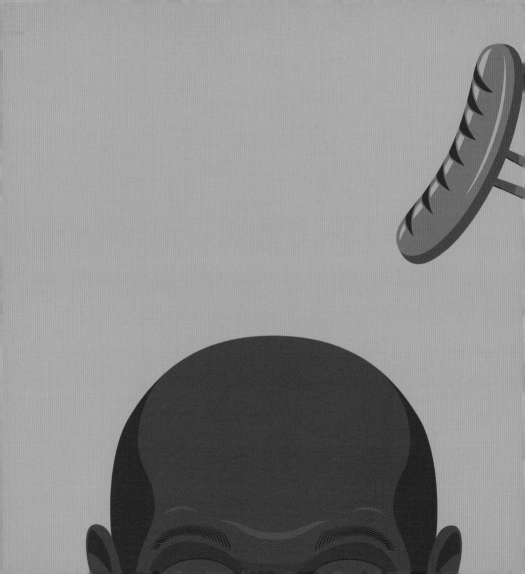

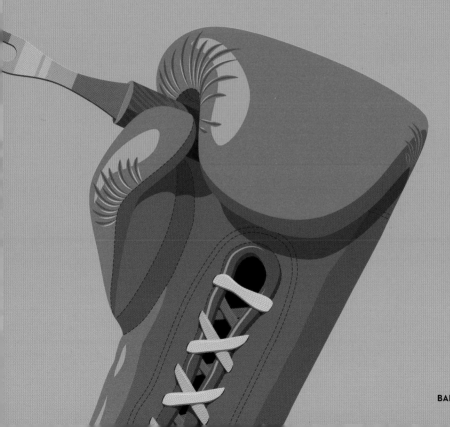

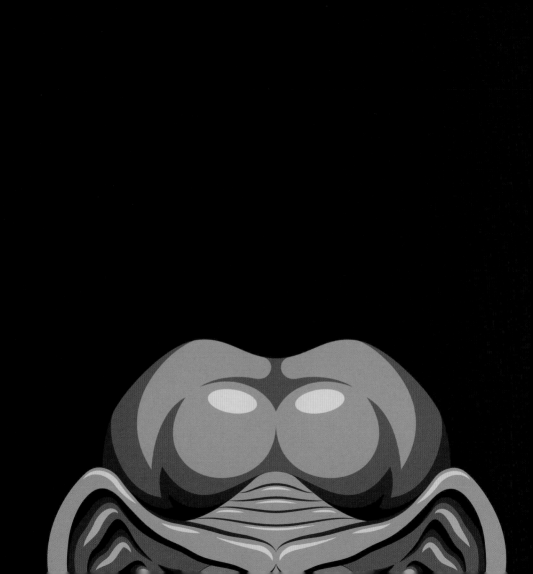

"All humans look alike."

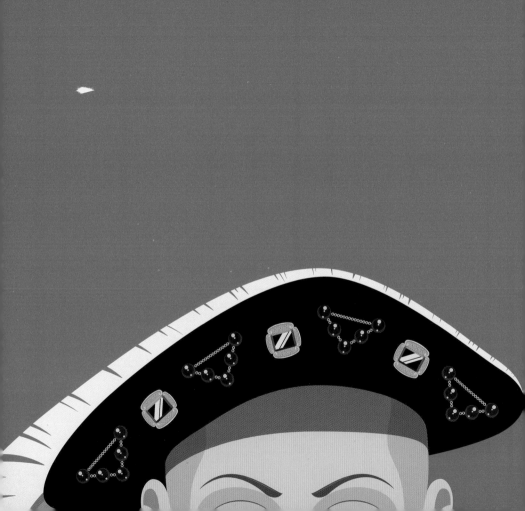

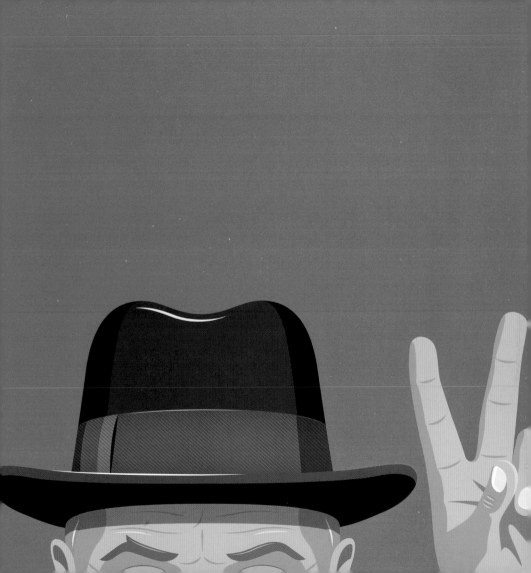

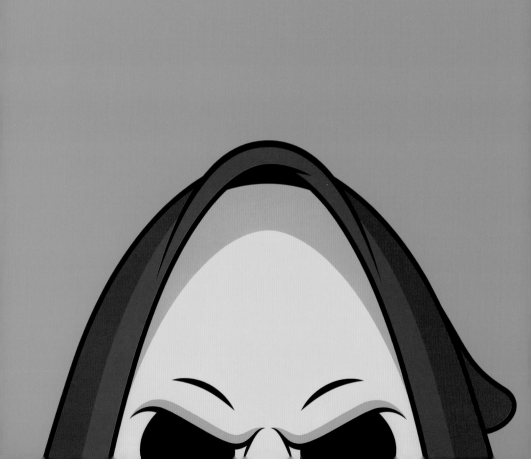

"Don't you ever feel like doing something evil?"

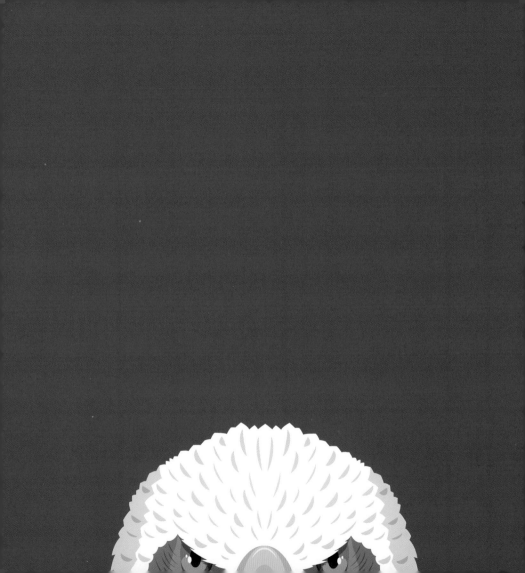

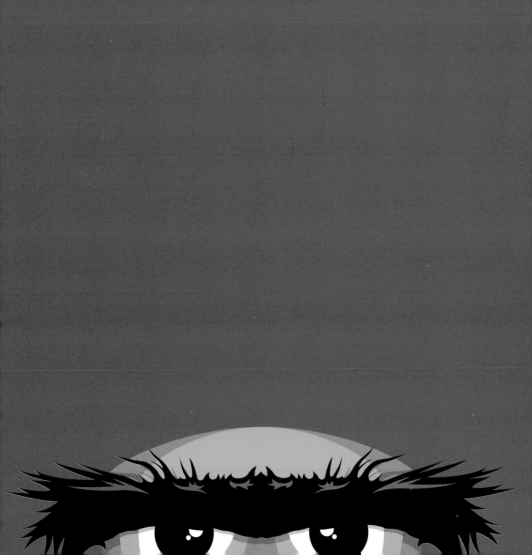

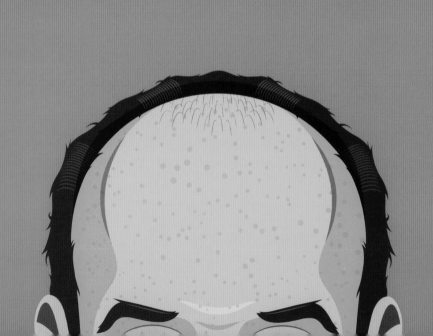

"Everything that's difficult you should be able to laugh about."

"Only I can live forever."

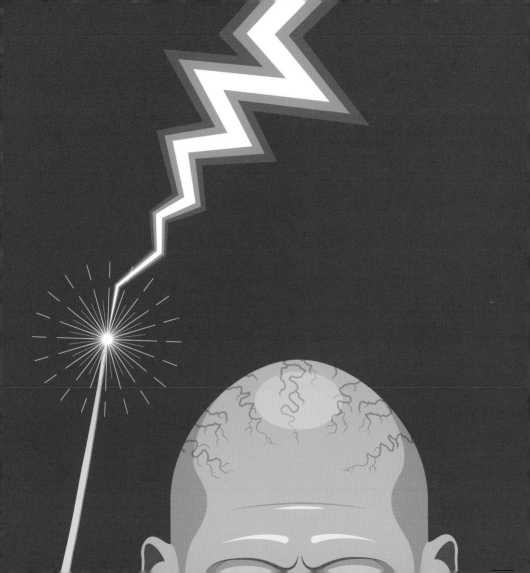

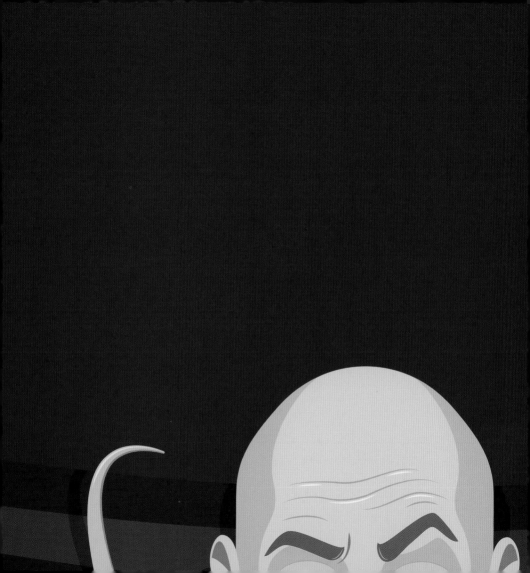

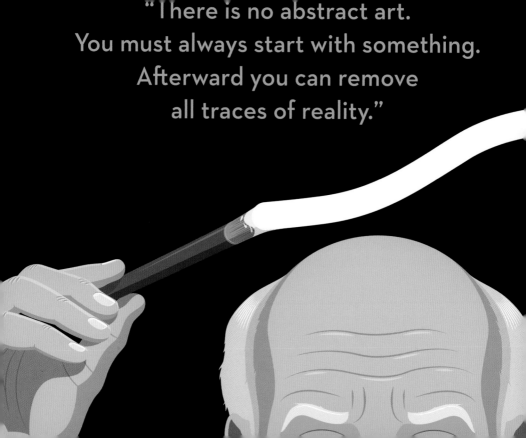

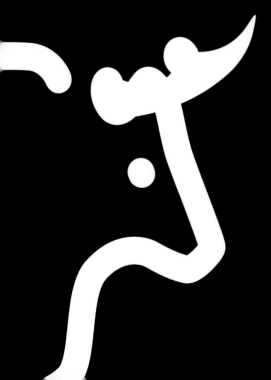

"Flame on!"

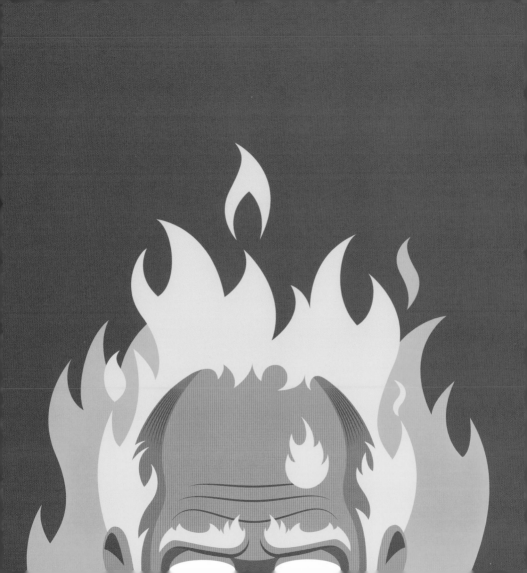

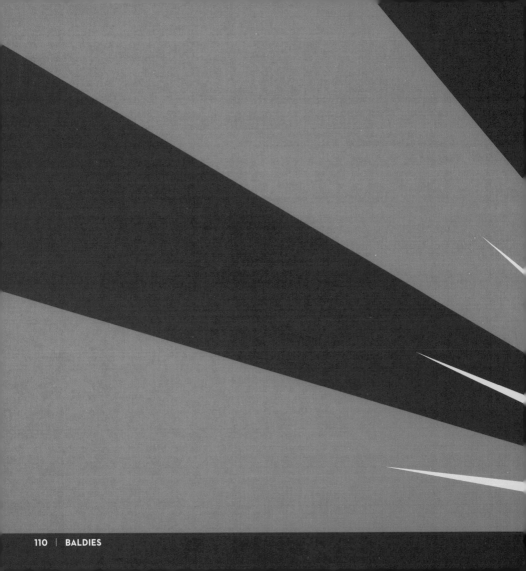

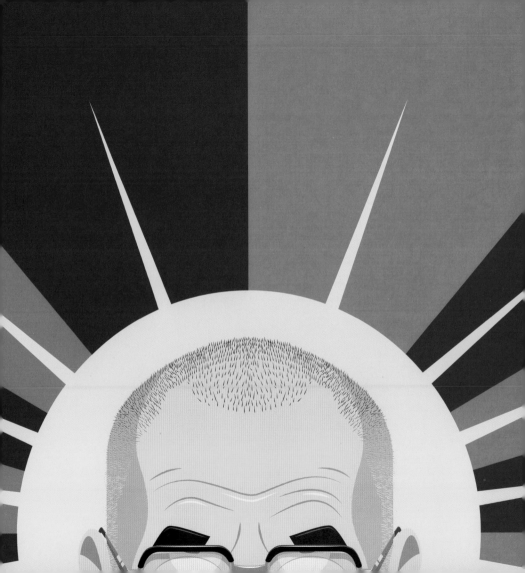

"There's power in pride!"

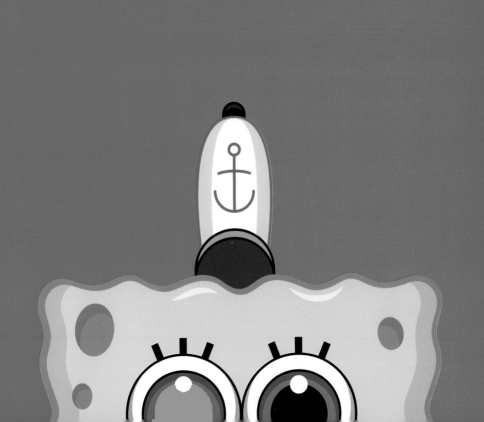

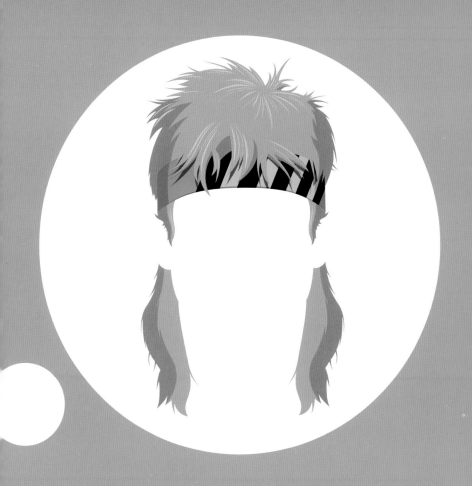

"Time is simultaneous, an intricately structured jewel that humans insist on viewing one edge at a time, when the whole design is visible in every facet."

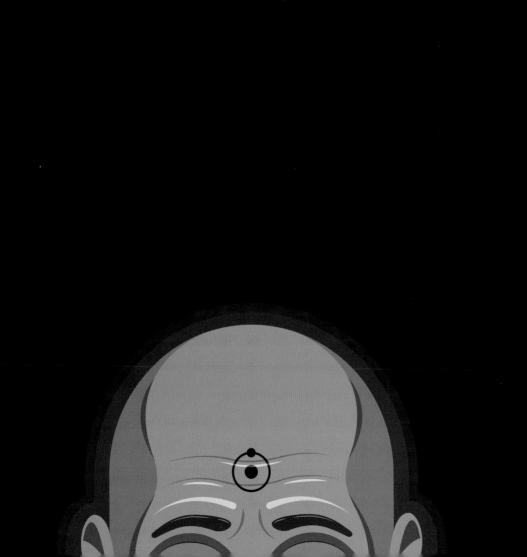

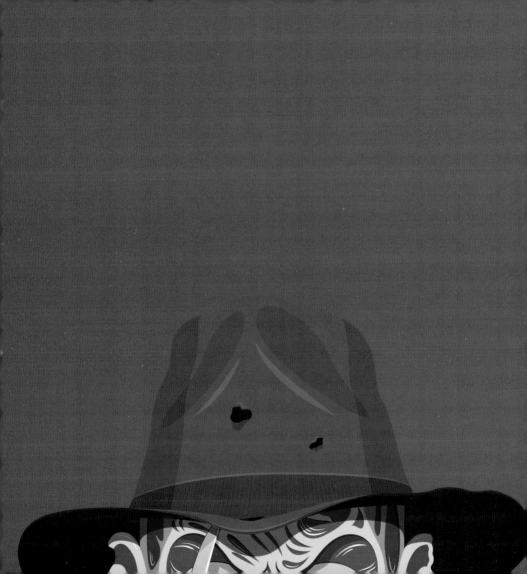

"Welcome to my nightmare."

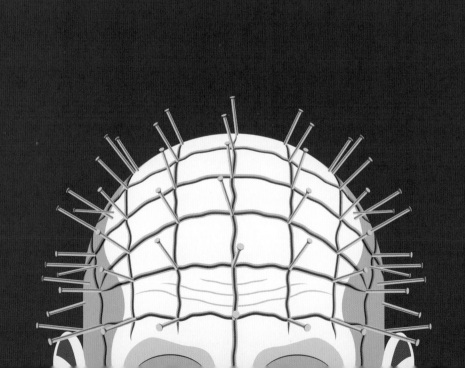

"Pain has a face.
Allow me to show it to you."

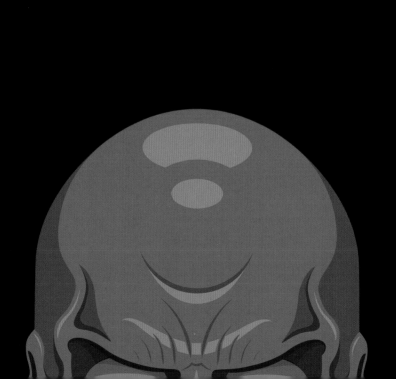

"You are deluded, Captain.
You pretend to be a simple soldier,
but in reality you are just afraid to admit
that we have left humanity behind.
Unlike you, I can embrace it
proudly. Without fear!"

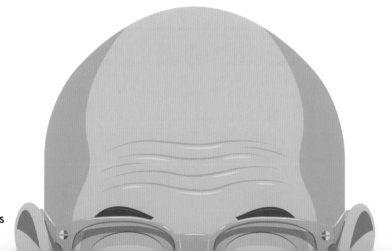

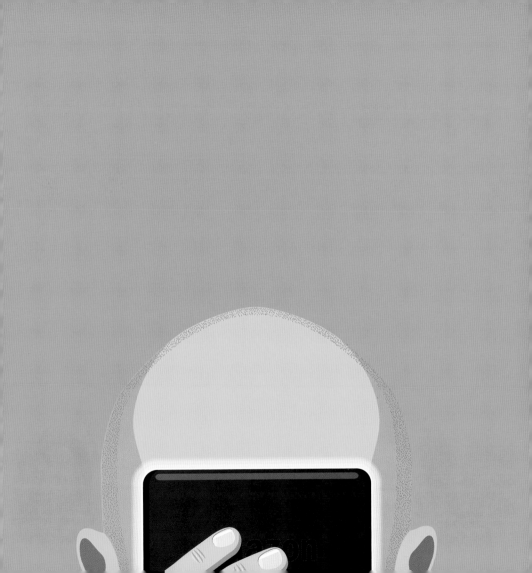

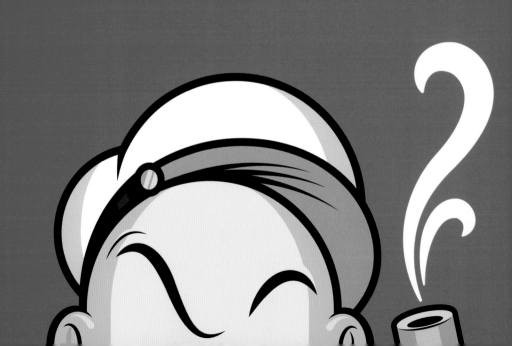

"Even though you're bigger than me, you can't win, 'cause you're bad, and the good always wins over the bad."

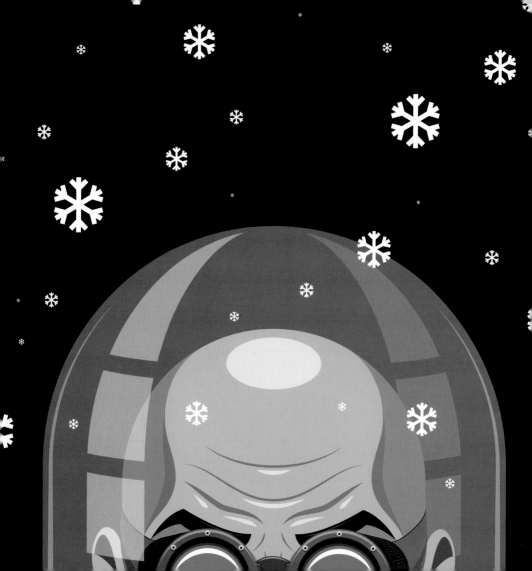

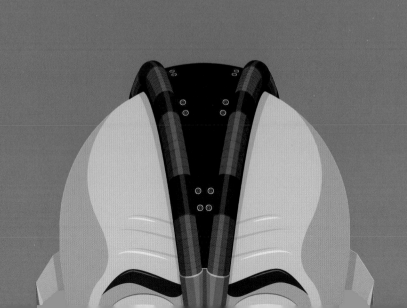

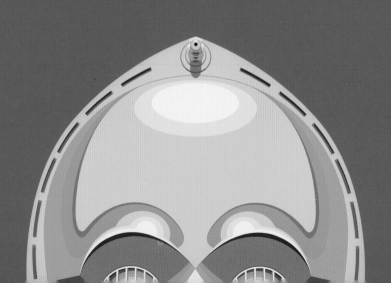

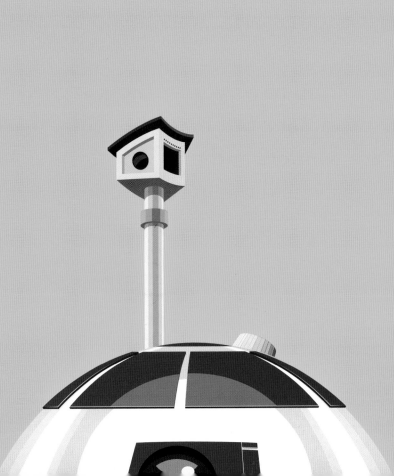

"You have been a most worthy adversary, but in every game, there are winners and there are losers. And as you know, in this game, losers get roboticized!"

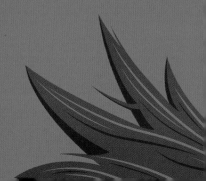

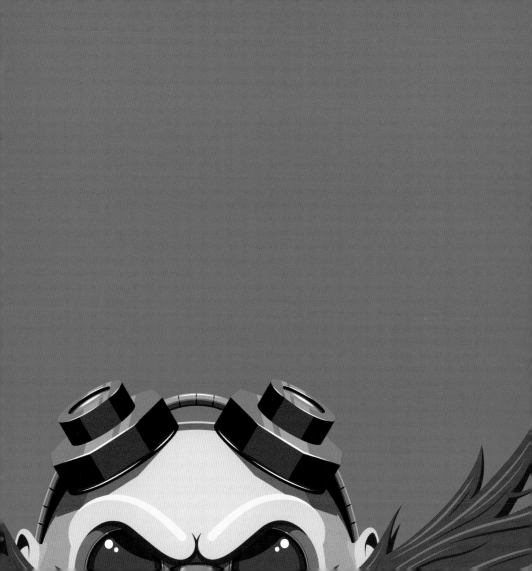

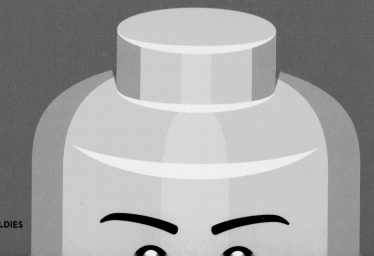

"To change the world we must be good to those who cannot repay us."

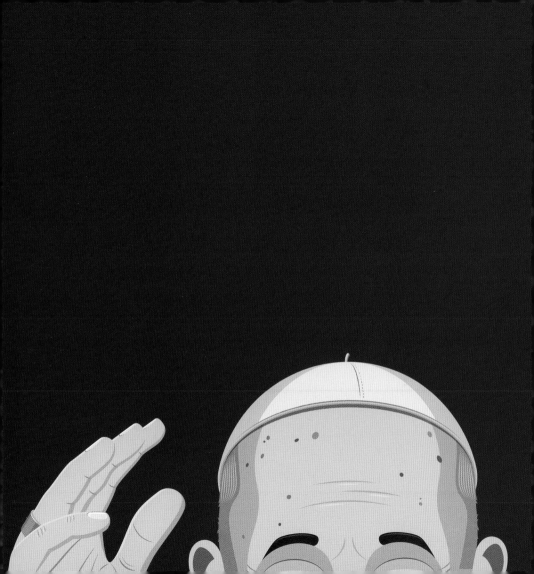

KEY

	pg. 2	Yoda		pg. 16	Shrek
	pg. 5	Homer Simpson		pg. 19	Dracula
	pg. 6	Nick Fury		pg. 20	Steve Jobs
	pg. 7	Samuel L. Jackson		pg. 22	Alien
	pg. 9	Kermit		pg. 23	Ellen Ripley
	pg. 10	Gandhi		pg. 24	Charlie Brown
	pg. 13	Professor X		pg. 27	Lex Luthor
	pgs. 14–15	The Blue Man Group		pg. 28	Mike Tyson

	pgs. 30–31	The Coneheads		pgs. 48–49	Michael Jordan
	pg. 33	Walter White		pg. 50	King Tut
	pg. 34	Stewie		pg. 51	Nefertiti
	pg. 36	Worf		pgs. 52–53	Dominic Toretto
	pg. 37	Jean-Luc Picard		pg. 55	The Mask
	pg. 38	Bender		pgs. 56–57	E.T.
	pg. 39	Professor Farnsworth		pg. 59	George Costanza
	pg. 40	Mr. Miyagi		pg. 60	Sloth
	pg. 42	Jackson Pollock		pg. 63	Darth Vader
	pg. 44	Predator		pg. 64	Hellboy
	pgs. 46–47	Gollum		pg. 67	Hunter S. Thompson

	pg. 68	Mr. Potato Head		pgs. 84–85	Shakespeare
	pg. 69	Buzz Lightyear		pg. 86	Robocop
	pg. 70	Larry David		pg. 89	Deadpool
	pg. 72	Gru		pgs. 90–91	George Foreman
	pg. 73	The Minions		pgs. 92–93	Quark
	pgs. 74–75	Furiosa		pg. 94	Henry VIII
	pg. 76	Mikhail Gorbachev		pg. 95	Winston Churchill
	pgs. 78–79	Morpheus		pg. 96	Skeletor
	pg. 80	Darth Maul		pg. 98	bald eagle
	pg. 81	The Night's King		pg. 99	Sam the Eagle
	pg. 82	Mr. Burns		pg. 100	Louis C.K.

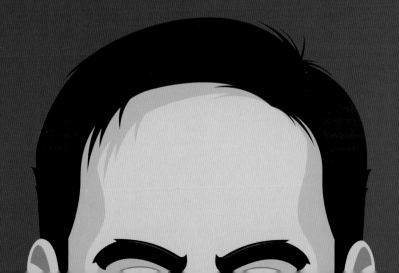

Fernando L. Perottoni is a
Brazilian illustrator, designer,
art director, entrepreneur, and
lasagna enthusiast, who, as you
can see, is not bald at all.
Yet.